My
Prostate Cancer
Adventure

and the

Lessons Learned

Craig Johnson

iUniverse, Inc.
Bloomington

iUniverse books may be ordered through booksellers or by contacting:

iUniverse
1663 Liberty Drive
Bloomington, IN 47403
www.iuniverse.com
1-800-Authors (1-800-288-4677)

ISBN: 978-1-4502-8206-2 (sc)
ISBN: 978-1-4502-8207-9 (ebook)

Printed in the United States of America

iUniverse rev. date: 01/13/2011

This book is dedicated to the

men and woman who have dedicated

their lives to understanding

cancers of all kinds.

Acknowledgments

First and foremost, I thank my wife, Maria, my companion over the last three decades, for her help in getting me through my recovery.

I also thank Brad Stern for his enthusiastic encouragement and support in making my recovery experiences available to other men contemplating prostate surgery.

And, lastly, many thanks to Susan Stern Bryson for her efforts in making my writing readable. I find it whimsically ironic that I required a woman's insight and humor to bring home my points about what is essentially a male problem.

Contents

PREFACE

On November 5, 2009, I underwent radical prostatectomy surgery in order to free myself from living with prostate cancer. Essentially everything in this book is based directly on my personal experiences before and after my prostatectomy. If you are planning to undergo another type of cancer treatment, your postoperative experiences may be very different from mine, and much of what I have to say about my recovery in the second half of this book may not apply to you.

When I was told that I had prostate cancer, my first thought was to find out what my options were. I didn't ask " Why me?" or begin wringing my hands about bad luck or attempt to apportion blame. None of those things would stop my cancer. Worrying only invites misery and often delays taking action, providing time for the cancer to grow and spread. I found myself in a bad situation, and I set out to deal with it.

In the first part of the book, I talk about how I came to the decision to undergo radical prostatectomy, and I describe my thoughts on the subject. My decision was based on my personal understanding of the therapies and treatments available at the time. Your decision should be based on your own careful consideration of the therapies available to you.

I am not a doctor, nor have I had medical training of any sort. Under no circumstances should the reader presume that I have expertise pertaining to any of the therapies I discuss in this book. I relied heavily on my urologist's suggestions and guidance. He gave me the basic information I needed to begin researching my condition and to reach a decision on how to deal with it.

I spent a lot of time searching the Internet and investigating the possibilities open to me. In addition, I searched out men who have had prostate cancer. I found that the men who have weathered this storm were eager to talk about their experiences when they realized that I was asking for myself. After all was said and done, I decided to go with a relatively new approach to prostate surgery: robotic prostatectomy.

Although I believe that my decision was the right one for me, this book is not an endorsement for robotic prostatectomy or any particular surgical procedure or therapy. My chief purpose in writing this book is to give the men who are considering radical prostatectomy a look at what they might expect during their own recoveries. The important thing to remember when dealing with cancer is that regardless of what you decide to do, your decision will come with consequences that will remain with you for the rest of your life. And so it is up to *YOU* to make the best choice that you can.

I urge the reader to consider the reasoning I present in this book as a sort of "devil's advocate" argument. Be critical of what I say and discuss your ideas with your doctor. By questioning everything I say in this book, you may gain a better understanding of the facts involved in your own situation.

Best of luck.

Craig Johnson

Introduction

The first thing the reader must know is that I am *not* a doctor. I have *zero* medical training. My only qualification for writing this book is that I have been through the experience of making the decisions that lead to selecting prostate surgery, as well as my experiences during postsurgical recovery.

I underwent a radical prostatectomy on November 5, 2009. The operation employed the use of a surgical robot guided by an experienced surgeon who was trained and certified to perform prostate surgery using the device.

About a week into my recovery, I was lying in bed, still a bit sore from the surgery, and it occurred to me that the next time I go through this I'll have an easier time of it. I'll know what to expect.

Then it occurred to me that I was all out of prostates!

And so I thought it would be a good idea to write my experiences down for the benefit of the guys who are considering prostatectomy surgery. This book is based *solely on my own experiences*. It is by no means a comprehensive list of recovery conditions or contingencies, but it might serve as a checklist of issues that you, your doctor, and others close to you can use to help you to come to a decision about how best to deal with your situation.

You may also want to keep this book handy during your own recovery as a kind of scorecard to compare your recovery with mine. (I did pretty well, but I hope you do better.) None of what's written here is rocket science. It's actually a lot of common sense, and it is likely that your doctor has already addressed much of what you'll read here. The difference between what the doctor tells you and what I put in this book is that the doctor is probably telling you his interpretation of what he's read and what his patients have told him about their recoveries. In this book, I'm providing the reader with a direct account of my own experience during my own recovery. I don't try to make one size fit everyone; this was how I came to the decision to undergo prostatectomy surgery and this was what it was like for me during my recovery.

I wrote this book in a very informal (some might even say vulgar) style. I wrote in about the same way I talk. I did this for two reasons. First, to remind you that I am not a medical expert and that everything I've written should be taken with a grain of salt. Second, my informal approach is to make you understand that what I have to say is the real deal. I'm not taking a clinical, ivory-tower approach here. I'm not attempting to convince you of what to buy or believe. This is me talking to you about something that has changed my life and how I've dealt with it.

I've made an effort to avoid names and places and not to recommend specific products I've used, but it should be pretty clear what I'm talking about.

No doubt there will be doctors who will take issue with what I say in this book. I've written this book from the patient's point of view – *my* point of view. There's bound to be disagreement between what I say here and the accepted medical consensus. When I was searching for information about prostate cancer, I found a lot of clinical information but relatively little information about how the patient felt and what the patient experienced. If nothing else, this book will make you think about the choices available to the prostate cancer patient. If you've decided on radical prostatectomy, as I did, you'll get some insight as to what to expect during your recovery.

The Adventure Begins

It was probably a sunny day in May 2009 when I paid a visit to my family doctor for my annual physical. It was almost certainly some time in the spring, because it was about six months after this visit that I underwent radical prostatectomy.

I was greeted by the usual receptionist, paid the usual co-payment, waited the usual amount of time that one waits when arriving on time at the doctor's office. And then I endured the usual poking and prodding that comes with an annual physical. About two weeks later, I paid the doctor a second visit to discuss the exam results. They were pretty much what I expected: need to lose some weight, blood pressure a little on the high side but normal, cholesterol is okay, vitamin D a little low, and, oh yes, my PSA score had jumped up to 4.7.

Hmm, okay. What do I do about it?

The doc slipped into what was obviously a well rehearsed monologue, the gist of which went like this: PSA stands for Prostate Specific Antigen, which is a substance that's made by the prostate. The "normal" amount can vary from person to person by quite a lot. My previous PSA scores were less than 1. This latest test was a very large jump from my norm.

"It could be nothing," said the doc. "There are men who have much higher PSA numbers who are living healthy lives."

A high PSA score might indicate an enlarged prostate, which happens to a lot to men in their mid-fifties. It might also be an indication of prostate cancer. He then said that everything seemed fine with my last digital rectal exam, so an enlarged prostate was not likely. I interpreted this as, *there's either nothing wrong with me or I have prostate cancer*!

Before I left the doctor's offices, the receptionist helped me to set up an appointment with an urologist.

The options of *I'm okay or I have cancer* didn't sit too well with me, so I started reading up about the whole PSA-prostate cancer thing on the Internet. It turned out that the PSA test isn't considered to be a very good indicator of prostate cancer. About a week later, I met this young urologist, let's just call him Dr. U. He seemed young to me, but then, ever since I hit fifty, a lot of people I meet seem young to me.

We engaged in the usual chit chat that strangers do when they're brought together in a room for the first time: "Nice weather we're having ... What do you do for living ... I'm an engineer ... How long have you been practicing ... Quite a while ... How many kids ... blah, blah, blah ..."

Before too long, the subject had turned to PSA tests and prostates. Dr. U pretty much repeated what my family doctor had said and also much of what I'd read about the PSA test—that it was not a good indicator of prostate cancer. There was a much better test for prostate cancer available. He wanted to conduct a prostate biopsy on me as soon as possible. I resisted his suggestion two reasons: first, the PSA test is not a reliable indicator of prostate cancer. I wanted a second PSA test to see if it would come up with similar results to the first test. For all I knew, the first test results were wrong, and this might be much ado about nothing. Dr. U insisted that a second PSA test was unnecessary. But I held firm, and he finally relented.

The second reason I wanted another PSA test was because I had read that, while the prostate biopsy was a much better indicator of prostate cancer than the PSA test, there were possible—not likely but possible—complications to a prostate biopsy, namely incontinence and erectile dysfunction. If I was to take on the risk of a prostate biopsy, I wanted to be damned sure there was a good reason to do so.

Before I left Dr. U's office he wanted to examine me himself. During the examination, he manually checked my testicles and penis. I suspect he was looking for signs of cancer or other disease. I didn't ask. The man was a professional; he knew his business. He then stuck his hand into a rubber glove and told me to turn around.

After the examination, he said in a matter-of-fact tone that everything appeared to be fine. Normally, I'd take some reassurance in that kind of statement, but I remembered what my family doctor left me thinking: there's either nothing wrong with me or I have prostate cancer. About a week later, I went to the lab to have blood taken for a second PSA test.

What Can You Say About PSA?

It turns out that the PSA test can predict cancer with about 30 percent accuracy. It's been argued that flipping a coin is a more reliable test, but that's not really true. Your prostate isn't flipping coins to pass the time. When the PSA number shoots up, *something* made it change. There are a number of things besides a swollen prostate and cancer that affect PSA blood levels.

Having sex one or two nights before a PSA test or a healthy bowel movement or even the doctor's digital rectal exam can bump up the PSA score.

Hmm ... did the doctor stick his finger up there *before* or *after* the nurse took my blood? I didn't remember. These came to be vitally important details to me, but none of which I questioned when blood was taken during my physical exam. But then, I didn't know anything about PSA test results at that time either.

Dr. U didn't see it the same way. He stressed that the next logical step was to perform a prostate biopsy, but I wasn't convinced. You see, I have what some people might think of as a jaded view of the medical profession. We like to think that doctors get into medicine because they want to save lives and be a benefit to society. And while that might be true for some in the profession, I don't put much faith in altruistic motivations when it comes to health-care professions. People become doctors for the same reason people become roofers, plumbers, lawyers or policemen—to earn a living.

Doctors get paid for each and every visit, and they get paid a little better if there's some kind of procedure associated with the visit.

And so, I made arrangements to have another PSA test performed. This time however, I would avoid everything within my control that would affect my PSA score during the three days prior to the blood test.

I had the second test performed and had the results sent to my family doctor. A few days later, I learned the results of the second test. They were not what I'd hoped for. My PSA test score was 4.2. While the number had actually dropped slightly, it had not dropped nearly enough. My PSA score used to be between 0 and 1. I had considered the possibility that the lab crew might have made a mistake in conducting the test, but twice in a row seemed to me very unlikely. So I went back to Dr. U and agreed to a prostate biopsy.

Dr. U reminded me that he had told me the second test wouldn't be useful and the results of the second test did seem to back up his opinion, but despite how the test turned out, I still disagreed with the good doctor. I've been an engineer most of my adult life. One of the fundamental aspects of engineering, or for that matter almost any other activity, concerns dealing with error. Some errors we can't avoid making, but we can take them into account.

Take measurement errors for example. Imagine that you need to cut a piece of wood to three feet, five and a half inches long. It seems pretty simple: get out the tape measure, run it along the selected piece of wood, and mark off three feet, five and a half inches. But when you mark the wood, how accurate are you going to be at that half-inch mark? Will you be a little to the right of the mark on the ruler or a little to the left? What about the width of the mark itself? Which edge of that mark, the right edge or the left, represents the actual three feet, five and a half inch length? Maybe you intend for the center of your mark to define the length—but then you have to "eye-ball" where that center is.

In order to deal with these types of errors, we establish tolerances. So now we can simply cut the wood three feet, five and a half inches, *plus or minus* an eighth of an inch. This saves a lot of grief. Never mind that the blade you're using to cut the wood has an eighth of an inch width with its own set of tolerances. As one might imagine, precision in measurement is at least as important in a medical lab as it is in a machine shop or lumber yard.

In my experience the most insidious type of error is human error. Even with established tolerances, a person can make a measurement error all too easily. Imagine doing the same test all day long, hour after hour. Isn't it reasonable to assume that somewhere along the line the person doing the testing is eventually going to make a mistake? What if that mistake is made while my PSA blood level is being tested? Supposing that a little too much of this sample is mixed with too little of that chemical agent? Or perhaps there's a calibration error in a device used in the measurement process? My point here is that when dealing with something as critically important as one's health, it is never unreasonable for a second test, especially if the risks involved in taking the test are low.

So was the second test useful? I think so. The consistently high PSA score proved to me that something was indeed going on with my prostate. Dr. U might have been convinced of this after seeing the results of the first PSA test, but then again, he's not the guy facing potentially bad news. With two out of two PSA tests yielding similar results, I was now ready to move on to the next logical step, the prostate biopsy.

Riding the Nail Gun

A prostate biopsy was the only way to tell if I had cancer or not. But even the prostate biopsy isn't 100 percent reliable. This is because during a biopsy, samples of cells are taken from the prostate and examined. It's entirely possible that this sampling can entirely miss whatever cancer cells are lying in wait in my prostate. The upshot of all this was that, if the results came back positive, then no shit, no kidding—I had cancer. But if the results came back negative, then I still *might* have cancer—the test just may not have picked it up because the biopsy sampling missed the cancerous cells.

What do you do if your biopsy results come back negative? You go on with your life, monitoring your PSA levels, and note any changes. You're also likely to have another biopsy every so often. Personally, I'd prefer to have a root canal.

Several weeks after I received my second PSA score, I prepared myself for the biopsy by taking antibiotics several days before the procedure. And in addition, a couple of Fleet enemas a few hours before I went to the doctor's office. Before long I found myself lying on my left side on a table in the doctor's operating room, facing a wall. I found the wall useful. It was something I could lean against with my right hand. I was wearing one of those flimsy paper robes that tie in back. The back was opened so that Dr. U could gain easy access to the area where he'd previously only stuck his gloved finger.

In the days prior to my prostate biopsy, I spoke with several guys who had been through it themselves. Almost all of them told me that it was a very uncomfortable experience. A couple of them said it was the worst thing they've ever endured. One guy told me it was a walk in the park, but then this same guy refuses Novocain or nitrous oxide when he sees his dentist. Needless to say I was somewhat concerned about the procedure I was about to undergo.

There are three basic ways a prostate biopsy can be performed. One involves a surgical procedure during which tissue is collected through a small incision. Another method uses something called a cystoscope, which is inserted through the urethra, like a catheter. The doctor is actually able to see inside the prostate and take a look around. I underwent the third, and I presume the most popular type of prostate biopsy, the transrectal biopsy. This involves a device called a biopsy gun, which uses spring-loaded needles to collect samples from the prostate. The doctor slides the gun into the rectum and fires needles, one at a time, through the rectum wall into the prostate. He uses an ultrasonic device to see where he's shooting. Thankfully, the good doctor provided local anesthetics to the area where he was working. It's ironic how one can be thankful for a shot in the ass.

The procedure didn't take very long, although for my part, it couldn't have ended soon enough. Dr. U took about a dozen samples, which seemed to go on forever. When he was done, I was surprised that I was able to get up off the table and get dressed. On the way out, I stopped at the reception desk to make a follow-up appointment. Then suddenly, I felt exhausted. I told the two nurses there that I couldn't believe that I actually had to pay to go on that ride. They giggled at that. I guess it was nice that somebody could laugh about it.

Seeing Red

After I finished the ride on the nail gun, Dr. U told me before I left his offices that I could expect to find blood in my stool, urine, and ejaculate over the course of the next two or three days. If the blood didn't start to fade within three days, I should let him know, and I should call him immediately if I started to feel very warm or hot, which would be an indication of infection.

It wasn't too long after I arrived home that the local anesthetic began to wear off and I was fairly sore for a couple of days after the biopsy to the point that I couldn't sit down. I stayed home from work the next day, but two days after the biopsy, I was back at work with a tolerably sore butt.

You know, it's one thing to be told what to expect, but it's quite another to actually experience pissing blood. Intellectually I knew this was only a temporary condition but between the pain and the bleeding from below, I have to admit I was beginning to get pretty depressed.

And the Winner Is …

A little more than a week later, I returned to the urologist's office to discuss the results of the biopsy. I suspected the doc would make a good poker player, because when I walked into his office I couldn't tell by looking at him if he had good news or bad news. Frankly, I was fairly certain, based on what I had read about PSA test results, that I didn't have prostate cancer. The odds were on my side—or so I thought.

I was disabused of that notion shortly after I sat down. Dr. U swung the computer monitor around on his desk so that I could see the display. He showed me pictures of the microscope slides containing the samples he'd taken during the biopsy. Most of the samples showed a nice uniform pattern of cells, all about the same size, nicely snuggled together. Then, he showed me two other slides that showed a few cells that were somewhat misshapen.

It looked pretty bad: the biopsy revealed the presence of cancer. I honestly have to say that I was more surprised than shocked or dismayed. There was less than a 30 percent chance that I had cancer based on the PSA test results, and yet there it was! I bought a couple of lottery tickets on the way back home that day.

I didn't win.

In my investigations, I had come across the interesting fact that prostate cancer is usually a slow growing cancer. The course of action taken in dealing with prostate cancer generally depends upon one's age, general health, and how advanced the cancer is. I was fifty-five when all this happened. If I had been seventy five, I very well might have decided not to have surgery. In fact, men in their seventies and eighties or older who are diagnosed with prostate cancer may feel compelled not to do anything about it at all. This is because there would be a good chance they won't be around long enough for the cancer to become a serious issue.

The Gleason Score

As such things go, I was relatively young to have prostate cancer. I probably owe it to the wholesome, healthy lifestyle of my younger days. Regardless of how I got it, I had it. And I had to figure out what to do about it.

Dr. U and I talked about my Gleason score, which provides an indication of how far along the cancer has progressed. Although I didn't know exactly how the Gleason score was derived (if you're interested, just ask your friendly urologist—he's probably been sitting around just waiting for someone to ask that very question) but it's pretty clear to me how it's used. The Gleason score ranges from 2 to 10. If your Gleason score is 4 or less, then you've likely caught the cancer in its early stages, or it's undetectable—if it's there at all. A score of 7 or higher indicates aggressive cancer activity. My Gleason score was 6, not terribly close to 4 and way too close to 7. The prognosis was that my cancer was most likely contained in the prostate and still not very aggressive.

I told Dr. U that I wanted a second opinion. Without hesitation he agreed and suggested a couple of clinical laboratories where the biopsy samples could be diagnosed. We decided on a lab, and he said he'd take care of it. As I said before, there's always the potential for human error. I felt that if two different labs come up with the same conclusions, the chances of human error being a factor in the diagnosis were greatly reduced.

Now, if I had been eighty years old and I had a Gleason score of 4, I'd probably thank the good doctor for his time, walk out his office, and not give the matter a second thought for the rest of my life. But I wasn't eighty years old. I was fifty-five, and I very much wanted someday to be eighty years old.

Dr. U gave me a lot of literature to read about the various therapies available for dealing with prostate cancer. We briefly discussed each of the available therapies, and he encouraged me to take my time to consider my options. We'd talk again in a few weeks. He suggested that I bring my wife at our next meeting in case she had questions.

Did You Hear The One About ...?

As I left the office, I thought about how I would broach the subject with my wife, Maria. We'd been married almost thirty years. This wasn't the first time she had to face a serious medical problem which concerned me. I had been involved in an automobile accident twenty-five years earlier that laid me up for three months. I woke up on a table with a lot of interns, doctors, and nurses hovering over me. I turned my head and saw Maria staring at me through a window. I thanked the people surrounding me, and told them that I'd have to leave now: my wife was here waiting for me. They all got a good laugh and told me I wasn't going anywhere. I had two broken legs, a broken arm, and a concussion. But that's a whole other story.

Then, there was the appendicitis attack about seven years ago. Once again, Maria caught up with me at the hospital. That time, I was on a gurney wearing one of those paper robes and freezing my butt off waiting for a CAT scan. She didn't say much. She just sat and stared at me the way she had after the car accident. They took my appendix out that evening, and I was discharged around noontime the next day. When Maria came by to take me home, she was her old self again.

This time around, I didn't have the ambiance of a hospital emergency room with which to broach the subject, so I did what I suppose most guys would do. I waited for her to bring it up. A few days later, she did.

"So, how'd your biopsy test come out?"

"Well," I said, "I have cancer."

"That's not funny," she scolded, annoyed that she wasn't getting a straight answer.

This was of course, my fault. I have a reputation for kidding around about very serious things, and I admit it. I'm probably one of the most irreverent people you'll ever meet. I make fun of politics, race, religion, handicapped people—you name it. If you can think of something that should be taken seriously, there's an excellent chance that I've already made a joke of it. No wonder she didn't believe me when I gave her a straight answer.

So, I turned and looked straight at her and said, "Yeah, I know it's not funny. I have prostate cancer."

Then, she gave me that look I saw twenty-five years ago when I was lying broken up on the table and years later when I was freezing my butt off on the gurney.

After a short silence, she said, "What are you gonna do?"

I wasn't sure yet. I used the literature that Dr. U provided to start my search for an answer to that question. As it turned out, there were a number of ways to deal with prostate cancer. They ranged from effectively doing nothing at all to bombarding the prostate with chemicals or hormones, to radiation (or a combination of those), to surgically removing the prostate and seminal glands, otherwise known as a radical prostatectomy. I was determined that the next time I went to see Dr. U that I would know exactly what I wanted to do, or I'd at least be able to discuss the matter from an informed standpoint.

Urologist, Myologist, Ourologist

Maria and I both took time off from work for the next visit to Dr. U. We had knocked some ideas around, but we hadn't come up with a definitive answer by that time. In addition to the material the doc gave me, I had been spending most of my free time reading all manner of material on the Internet about the various treatments available for prostate cancer.

You have to be careful about what you read on the Internet. I tried to stick to clinical websites, medical journals, support group websites for prostate cancer patients, and the like. There's a lot of great information available on the web, but there are also a lot of crackpots out there with websites designed specifically to separate you from your money. These websites are the modern-day snake-oil salesmen, touting vitamin formulas to ward off or cure all sorts of disease, diet plans, magnetic rings, crystals, and aroma therapies. They rely on the fear and desperation of people confronted with misfortune. I preferred to stick to the websites with established scientific credentials.

Maria and I were making this visit to find out what the second opinion was on my biopsy and also so that Maria could hear for herself what the doc had to say.

Dr. U greeted us warmly, and we all sat down around his desk. He came to the point quickly; the second diagnosis confirmed the first. There was no doubt about it. I had prostate cancer. The good news is that I was young, in good health, and there was a very good chance that I could be cancer free within a month or two. The doctor explained everything to Maria that he'd previously explained to me. Of course, none of this was news to Maria, as I'd told her all this myself. And, in addition to what she heard from me, she almost immediately started her own investigation into the matter using the Internet after I had told her that I had cancer.

Dr. U was a surgeon; he recommended radical prostatectomy. If the cancer was localized to the prostate as he suspected, there was an excellent chance that removing the prostate would cure me of the disease for the rest of my life, but he didn't want us to make a decision right there and then. He wanted us to talk to each other about it and come see him in a few weeks. I didn't tell the doctor that I was already near a decision. At that time, I was learning more about the various therapies available to me, and I was leaning toward either radiation therapy or robotic radical prostatectomy. (I go into more detail about my thoughts on surgery and therapies later in the book). Dr. U handled prostate cancer the old-fashioned way, by manually performing prostatectomies. By now, I was certain that I did not want this approach, which meant that I would not be making use of Dr. U's surgical skills, but I decided to keep this to myself until I had made a final decision.

So What Do I Do Now?

There is no one right answer to this question. One size does not fit all. At the very least, it is a deeply personal question whose answer will impact the life of the cancer victim as well as the lives of his family for as long as they're together. In my humble opinion, selecting a course of action in dealing with prostate cancer should not be a rushed decision—unless of course, you're confronted with an aggressive cancer problem.

As I saw it, this thing had been growing inside me since before my last physical a year earlier. Taking a few more weeks to consider my options was unlikely to make much of a difference. To start, my decision depended on a number of things in addition to age, general health, and how advanced the cancer was. There was also the quality of life issue. Certainly, I had to consider the immediate effects of the procedure I chose, but the long-term effects of my decision were most important. What would be the implications for Maria and me, and how would *we* live with the results for the rest of our lives?

I was lucky in that I was in a good position to consider and choose how I would deal with my disease. Pretty much all the possible options for beating this thing were on the table for me: watchful waiting, chemotherapy, cryotherapy, hormonal therapy, radiation therapy, and radical prostatectomy.

Although I will briefly discuss each of these therapies in this book, I certainly cannot explain them any better than your doctor. My intent in this book is to let you, the reader, know what was going through my mind when I made the decisions I made. If, after reading this book, you think that I've made mistakes along the way, then good! You won't make the same mistakes that I made. Just be sure to discuss all of these therapies with your doctor before you make *your* decision.

Back to the subject at hand ...

After learning something about each of the methods used to treat prostate cancer, it struck me that most of my options would have detrimental effects on the healthy parts of my body not infected with cancer. The popular impression is that healthy, non-cancerous cells can recover from treatment with relative ease, while cancerous tissues will tend to wither and die off. I had a hard time believing that cancer cells are so fragile that they can be killed off without seriously affecting healthy tissues in the process.

Take chemotherapy for example. There are a number of ways of taking chemotreatment. They range from sitting in a clinic and getting toxic chemicals injected into the body to taking a pill at home one or more times a day. I didn't like this approach because the medication damages healthy cells as well as the targeted cancer cells. Presumably, it doesn't kill healthy cells as easily as the cancerous ones, but I couldn't see that it did healthy cells any good, either. Here's the part that I really didn't like: the medication runs through your *entire* body—heart, brain, kidneys, liver, spleen—you name the organ, the toxin is going to stream through all parts of your body. As I understood it, chemotherapy is generally reserved for guys suffering from advanced stages of cancer and under situations in which the cancer has spread beyond the prostate itself. Fortunately for me, my cancer appeared to be confined to my prostate, so I could scratch chemo off my list of possible therapies.

Hormonal therapy works to decrease the level of testosterone in the prostate. One form of hormonal therapy, orchiectomy, is actually a fancy word for removing the testes. Just as with chemotherapy, the medications used in hormone therapy circulate throughout the entire body. I wasn't a candidate for hormone therapy because the procedure is generally used for guys with higher Gleason scores than I had. I said earlier that I was lucky. I was certainly lucky enough to have avoided castration! I took hormone therapy off my list with a sigh of relief.

Radiation therapy covers two basic approaches for dealing with the disease. There are internal methods, and there are variations of external radiation treatment. From the stuff I read, it seemed to me that proponents of radiation therapy like to make the case that radiation can be focused directly onto the prostate, giving the impression that the prostate is the only part of the body that's affected by the radiation. It would be nice if that were true, but I didn't buy it.

One form of radiation therapy involves seed implants; these are little, radioactive bits that are surgically placed into the prostate. The idea is that the radiation spewing out of these seeds is intense enough to kill nearby cancer cells. But it seemed to me that this method suffers from some of the same problems as chemotherapy—any form of radiation that can kill cancer cells can kill healthy tissue as well. Or so it seems to me. I mean, how's a gamma ray supposed to know the difference between good and bad cells? And consider this: the radiation pouring out of those seeds doesn't just stop at the cancer cell; it moves right along through all the other tissues in its path until it leaves the body. It then keeps on going in a straight line forever or until it gets absorbed by something, like a piece of heavy metal. The point here is that not only do seeds destroy cancer cells in the prostate, they can also do damage to much of the surrounding tissues in the bladder, rectum, etc. In fact, guys who opt for seed therapy are advised not to let children, pets, and other living things sit in their laps, lest they get a dose of radiation.

External radiation is another effective method for dealing with prostate cancer, but it suffers from similar side effects of radioactive seeds. Sure, "beams of radiation" are focused from *outside* your body onto your prostate, but in order to get *to* your prostate, the beams must travel *through* the healthy tissues of your body. I had a hard time believing that these beams can be focused through living tissue so precisely so as to affect only prostate cells. It seemed to me that, just as with the radioactive seed method, the surrounding healthy tissue must also be adversely affected.

Now, maybe I'd seen too many B-grade science fiction flicks from the fifties, but radiation not only acts to destroy living tissue, there's the prospect of mutating cells in living tissue as well. In killing off the original prostate cancer, isn't there the potential for causing new cancers to form? Does this really happen? Probably not in the short term, but what about the long-term potential, ten or twenty years down the road? I suppose this isn't a source of concern if you're in your seventies or eighties, but I was fifty five when I was diagnosed and I wanted to cure myself of prostate cancer. I didn't want to lay the groundwork for another cancer to take hold years later.

One last thing about radiation, hormone, and chemo therapies: if these procedures don't completely destroy all of the cancer, or if new cancer should emerge after some period of time, surgery to correct the situation in most cases is difficult or impossible. At least, this was my understanding when I was investigating my options.

Consider this: If I had decided to go the radiation route only to find out that it didn't "take," I would still have prostate cancer and a surgical solution might very well be out of the question. This would mean living with cancer and possibly subjecting myself to periodic chemotherapy or hormone treatments for the rest of my life.

Although I took radiation therapy off my list, you should definitely discuss the various radiation therapies in detail with your doctor before you make the same decision. Times change and technologies improve.

This brings us to cryotherapy, a cool-sounding way to get rid of prostate cancer. Cryotherapy is a relatively new procedure that uses intense cold to kill cancer cells. At the time I was diagnosed, I couldn't find a lot of reliable information on this procedure. It seemed to me that the chief proponents of cryotherapy are the people who want to *develop* cryotherapy. One good thing about cryotherapy is that if the first attempts to kill off the cancer aren't successful, other cryotherapy attempts can be made. That, in my humble opinion was the only thing in this procedure's favor. In the material I found on cryotherapy, incontinence and impotence could easily result from the procedure. But then, the risk of incontinence and impotence was a possibility from all the methods of treating prostate cancer that I've read about. Frankly, I'm not in a hurry to become a test case for medical experimentation, so I scratched cryotherapy off my list.

Don't Be Such a Wimp

You might say, "So what if there's a little collateral damage? You want to kill cancer? These therapies will kill it. Who really cares if there are unintended casualties in the area?"

In answer to that question, consider the prostate's neighborhood— what else lives in the general area?

First of all, there's the major business area of the rectum. Killing off tissues down there could affect one's ability to move the bowels. The urinary bladder is another one of the prostate's next-door neighbors. Killing off tissues in and around the bladder can lead to incontinence. There are also important nerves and blood vessels in the immediate area which help to control and nourish tissues needed to gain and maintain an erection.

All the therapies I've talked about so far have consequences to varying degrees concerning incontinence and impotence. I was in no hurry to live the remainder of my life wearing a diaper, and even at the ripe old age of fifty five, I know I'd miss getting a boner.

Keep in mind that, at the time I was faced with making this decision, the state of the art of these therapies hadn't reached a level of precision that I was comfortable enough to use. Radiation, chemo, cryo, and hormonal therapies all aim at the prostate, but the way I saw it, their effect was less like a rifle and more like a shotgun. Tissues all throughout the surrounding area of the prostate, or throughout the body in general were likely to be adversely affected. Having said this, with the rapid development of medical technologies today, it is all important to conduct your own investigation into each of these and other newer therapies that might emerge.

After considering and discounting the various ways of dealing with my problem I was left with two methods of dealing with prostate cancer still on my list: watchful waiting and prostatectomy.

Watchful waiting is just that—your doctor monitors the progression of your cancer with periodic PSA tests and digital rectal exams. I seriously considered this for a while. After all, my cancer was apparently slow growing and in its early stages. I might have been able to put off doing anything about it for a few more years. If and when the cancer became a major problem, I could decide on a course of action at that time.

The advantage to this approach was that I could just go on with my life until the cancer became a more serious issue. Hell, I didn't even know I had cancer until my biopsy results came in. Up to that time, I felt just fine. Other potential advantages of watchful waiting were that medical technologies would likely advance and that the precision in dealing with the cancer might be much improved.

The disadvantage, however, was that in 2008 there was no indication that I had prostate cancer; then, the very next year BOOM! I'm diagnosed with cancer with a Gleason score of 6. While it's true that I might have been able to put off undergoing cancer treatment for a few years, I'd be living those years knowing that I had a growing cancer in my body. This was not something I took lightly. Cancer is not really isolated by organ boundaries from all other cells. They all drink from the same glass—the circulatory and lymphatic systems that connect our organs. Whatever it is that makes prostate cells cancerous might make its way outside the prostate and start wreaking havoc in other tissues. I'm certainly no oncologist, but we've all heard that cancer can spread and that thought was at the forefront of my thinking.

Maybe I sound a bit paranoid, but it's hard not to be paranoid when you're dealing with cancer. Nonetheless, I left watchful waiting on my list, for a little while anyway.

Prostatectomy was the last thing I considered, and it turned out to be the procedure I decided to use.

There are generally two flavors of radical prostatectomy: robotic/laparoscopic and, for lack of a better term, "traditional" prostatectomy.

Traditional prostatectomy involves making an incision, ten or more inches long, below the navel. The surgeon then removes the prostate and seminal glands. During the course of the surgery, it is entirely possible (in my mind, it was entirely *likely*) that the surgeon can damage the nerves and blood supply that support the functions of the urinary bladder and penis. There is a "nerve-sparing" technique in which the surgeon makes the attempt not to damage nerves that affect one's ability to control urine flow and erections.

While reading about this surgery, I thought it was a bit weird that writers went through the trouble of describing prostatectomy surgery and *then* included a few sentences that said something like,

"Oh yes! There's also the new nerve-sparing technique!" It's almost as though they thought a guy would actually consider *not* selecting the nerve-sparing technique.

To me, the traditional surgery solution with the nerve-sparing technique seemed better than the other therapies. Clearly, the surgeon has much tighter control using a scalpel during surgery than the chemical, hormones or radiation methods offered.

Enter my concerns of human error. Certainly, the surgeon I chose for the job would have performed the surgery hundreds, maybe thousands, of times. I wanted no beginners in my innards. But even experienced surgeons can make mistakes. If I were to undergo surgery, I wanted to get the risk of a mistake as low as it could possibly get. That's where robotic surgery came in.

Robotic surgery seemed to me to be the solution of choice, and here's why: instead of a single large incision, a number of small incisions are made to provide the robotic arms access inside the body. Less of my insides would be exposed to the open air, and presumably, this would mean a lower risk of infection. The surgeon has a *very* close-up, high-definition, full-color view of what he's doing during surgery with the robotic approach and exquisite precision over the surgical tools used.

The surgery is performed from a console equipped with a high-definition, binocular monitor system, which gives the surgeon a three-dimensional view. The robot itself has a number of "arms," each of which has a special tool at its end, one of which is a high-definition video camera. The surgeon is able to perform the surgery almost as if he were standing right next to the prostate. Nerve-sparing procedures in robotic surgery are managed not at arms' length, but with the precision of the robotic end effectors (tools), and a well lit, close up 3D view of all the action in the area. I found video clips on the Internet that showed the surgeon's view of an actual prostatectomy surgery being performed. I was impressed with the precision with which the surgeon could control the robotic tools inside the patient. As to recovery time, patients are often out of the hospital the next day, but the surgery requires several weeks of at-home recovery.

As I saw it, the surgical approach greatly reduced the possibility of collateral damage with respect to the surrounding tissues, and robotic prostatectomy had the advantages of small incisions, short hospital stay, low risk of losing bowel and urinary control, and a relatively low risk of impotence. In addition, if somehow the surgeon didn't get all the cancer out, I still had recourse to additional surgery or the other available therapies. This isn't always the case with the non-surgical alternatives. I had convinced myself that robotic prostatectomy was the way to go, and so I set out to talk to guys who had undergone robotic prostatectomy to find out what they thought of it.

Chances Are One Out of Six

It's said that one out of every six men are destined to deal with prostate cancer. Personally, I find that to be an amazing statistic. So amazing in fact, that I didn't believe it at first. And yet, all I had to do was mention prostatectomy at my job, and almost immediately, I had references to four guys who have actually had the surgery performed. And after talking to these first four, all of whom I personally knew at work, I learned of several more guys outside of work. In fact, my wife Maria has a close family member who has had a prostatectomy—someone I'd known for years, but I didn't find out about his prostatectomy until I brought up the subject.

Men diagnosed with prostate cancer should not be embarrassed or ashamed of it. Prostate cancer is not a disease you get by sitting on a dirty toilet seat or cavorting with unsavory types. It's not contagious. However you got it, you got it honestly.

Actually, no one really knows what exactly causes prostate cancer. There are however, some factors which appear to contribute to the onset of the disease:

- Age (usually fifty years and older)
- Genetics (apparently inherited from your father's side)
- Diet (animal fat seems to play a role)
- Testosterone (feeds the growth of cancer cells)

The point here is if you're diagnosed with prostate cancer there is an excellent chance that you can find someone to talk to about it. Keeping quiet about your condition may work more against you than for you.

Lesson Learned: don't go it alone! If you're diagnosed with prostate cancer and want to discuss it with someone who's been through it, ask almost anyone. There is a very good chance that someone you know either has it, has had treatment for it, or knows someone who has been through the experience.

Thank You, But No Thank You

After deciding upon robotic/laparoscopic surgery to treat my cancer, I went back to Dr. U to give him the bad news. It was bad news for him because he was a traditional surgeon who wasn't trained in robotic surgery. I entered his office expecting an argument. Dr. U had introduced me to the therapies available, and he indicated early on that he believed that radical prostatectomy was the way to go. But now that I agreed with him, I decided it wasn't going to be him to perform the surgery.

When I told him about my decision, he took it far better than I thought he would. He nodded in agreement and asked me if I had a surgeon in mind. As a matter of fact I did. It was the same surgeon who had treated a couple of the guys I interviewed. They both felt fine, and they had nothing but good things to say about the guy. In fact, I already had an appointment to meet with the surgeon later the same week.

Dr. U agreed that robotic prostatectomy was the hot new thing in prostate cancer, and it showed a lot promise. We shook hands. He gave me his card and told me not to hesitate to call him if I had any questions or problems after the surgery. I left his office feeling pretty good. Perhaps my view of the medical profession was a bit too cynical after all.

Meeting the Robot Surgeon

The ride to meet the surgeon took about thirty minutes. Because I don't have permission to use his name I'll refer to him as Dr. S. The guys who referred me to this doctor thought he was the greatest thing since sliced bread.

As I sat in Dr. S's waiting room, I started up a conversation with a gentleman sitting right across from me. It turned out that Dr. S recently performed radical prostatectomy on him, and he had the same praise for the surgeon as the guys I spoke with earlier. I was impressed. I asked him how the recovery went; he said that he was still recovering. The first couple of weeks were tough, but he was coming along fine. When he was called into the doctor's office I noticed that he rose slowly from his chair and walked carefully to the office door. Another guy overheard our conversation and agreed with the first guy. *Not bad,* I thought: two unsolicited endorsements from two patients right there in the waiting room.

About fifteen minutes later, the gentleman I first spoke to came walking out. His movements were a bit slow, but he had a big smile on his face. He gave me a thumbs up as he proceeded down the hallway. The receptionist called my name.

A nurse showed me to a small examination room and told me that the doctor will be in to see me shortly. A few minutes later, Dr. S came in and introduced himself. He looked as if he had just stepped right out of a soap opera. He was a handsome young doctor, and he stood about five foot ten or eleven and had a dark complexion. He told me was from India, although I could discern no trace of an accent. Have you ever seen a person who exudes confidence? One glance at this guy and you *knew* he had his shit together.

The meeting was pretty much what you'd expect. He told me about himself; I told him about myself. How'd I find out about him? I said, a couple of guys from work, and I told him their names. He remembered one of the guys pretty clearly. It seemed that the illustrious Dr. S does a lot of surgeries each week, so it wasn't surprising that he wouldn't remember everyone he'd worked on. He told me that he held surgery on Tuesdays and Thursdays. He said that, at the time I met him, he had performed over nine-hundred prostatectomies.

He went on to explain that the surgery usually lasts about three hours, give or take. We went over my medical history, and then he went into some detail describing the radical prostatectomy surgery. I asked if he needed to take everything—the prostate and the seminal glands—or could he just remove the affected parts of the prostate?

No, he told me. They take it all out, and the urethra is cut when the prostate is removed but it is then reattached.

I asked about incontinence and impotence. He asked me if I had trouble getting an erection. Well, no, I replied—I still had my towel hanger.

He smiled at that. That was another thing: this doctor didn't talk down to me like doctors seem to talk down to their patients. I think there must be a course in medical school, Patronizing the Patient 101, required for anyone who wants to have a bunch of letters after their name. Dr. S's demeanor was easy going and casual. We talked as if we'd known each other for years. I felt completely at ease.

He told me that, out of all his patients, three were dealing with incontinence problems. As it happens, all three were also very much overweight. I don't think he used the word *obese*, but he certainly implied it. He explained that men grow up naturally depending on the prostate to help regulate urine flow. After undergoing a prostatectomy, that safety valve is no longer there. Women aren't born with prostates, they rely on the sphincter muscle at the base of the urinary bladder and pelvic floor muscles to control urine flow. After the surgery, I'd have to work at developing control over these same muscles to avoid incontinence. In short, after the surgery and for the rest of my life I'd be pissing like a girl, only I'd be standing up while doing it.

I would have to start doing Kegel exercises to help strengthen the pelvic floor muscles, a major requirement in avoiding incontinence. Overweight men put more pressure on the bladder than average-sized guys. This can cause problems in regulating urine flow, especially when the prostate is no longer around to act as a safety valve.

As far as erections were concerned, few men get through prostatectomy surgery with the ability to get an erection right away. It can take months, a year, or more in some cases to recover, and even then, a full recovery in overall size is never guaranteed.

Then there's the matter of baby making. Radical prostatectomy pretty much makes this a thing of the past. The prostate serves as sort of a staging area for ejaculation. It's where semen and sperm get together prior to their launch into the great unknown. Without seminal glands and a prostate, sperm have no way to get out of the body. The testicles will still provide testosterone and make the little swimmers, but the pool's been removed and so the little wigglies are absorbed back into the body.

With those sobering thoughts, the good doctor gave me more stuff to read and requested that I ask my family doctor to forward my medical records to his office. Just before I left, he had to perform a digital exam to check my prostate. I guess he wanted to make sure I still had one before he agreed to perform the surgery. It occurred to me a forefinger up the butt is the urologist's version of shaking hands.

Goin' for It

I read the material Dr. S gave me. It agreed with everything I had already read and everything he had told me during our first meeting. Still, I was hesitant to make a commitment to surgery. This wouldn't simply be a big step in my life. It would be a life-changing event.

No matter how good the surgeon is, there is always a risk with surgery.

I asked Dr. S about the possibility of contracting MRSA while I was in surgery or in recovery. He assured me that MRSA can be a concern in the sick ward, but it was not a concern in the operating room or in surgical recovery.

In case you didn't know, MSRA stands for Methicillin-Resistant Staphylococcus Aureus (I got that from the Internet). I've heard of people who have contracted MRSA (pronounced *MERSA*) during their stay in hospital. It seems that this little nasty is everywhere: on shopping cart handles, restroom doors, and especially in hospitals. Apparently, most people are immune to it, but if it gets into your blood, it can become a problem. The last thing I needed was to undergo cancer surgery only to wind up riddled with an incurable staph infection. The best way to prevent MRSA from becoming a problem is simple—use good hand hygiene. Wash your hands four times a day to keep the MRSA away.

Over the course of my life, as I suspect is true with most people, I've been too cautious about some decisions and not cautious enough about others. The decision I was now contemplating would ultimately be a factor in deciding how long I lived, as well as how well I lived. Frankly, the thought that I might wind up wearing a diaper for the rest of my life was enough for me to reconsider watchful waiting. I discussed my concerns with some of the guys who had gone through the robotic procedure. All of them dismissed my apprehensions flat out. The first two months will be the toughest, they agreed. After that, you begin to get your control back. I walked away convinced that robotic prostatectomy was the way to go. I must admit that Dr. S was very successful in assuaging my cynical disposition concerning surgeons' motivations. I was very impressed with Dr. S, and the guys I'd talked to all seemed to have come through the surgery none the worse for wear.

I called Dr. S's office and made an appointment for surgery.

The Big Day

After I made the appointment the days seemed to fast forward to November 5, 2009. Some two weeks before the surgery, I began having trouble sleeping through the night. I didn't *feel* especially nervous about the surgery, at least not consciously, but I was thinking about it every day.

As we drove to the hospital on the big day, Maria didn't appear to be especially nervous, but she was obviously annoyed at having to be at the hospital so freakin' early in the morning. Maria's not a morning person. As for me, I intended to sleep the whole day through—starting at the time when they stuck that needle in me on the cutting board. I just wanted to get it over with and get it behind me.

As is probably the norm with most hospitals when arriving on time for surgery, we checked in at the reception desk and were then told to wait. I guess we sat around for about forty minutes before they sent us into an examination room, where we waited some more. About fifteen or twenty minutes later, a nurse came by to ask me a bunch of questions about how I was feeling and about my medical history.

Did they even look at my medical records?

She asked if I'd had anything to eat since going to bed. I set her mind at ease. Nothing since dinner, not even coffee. I signed some papers, which I'm sure would somehow make me legally responsible in the event that anything went wrong during the surgery. After all, a problem in the O.R. would *have* to be my fault as I'd be the only person in the operating room without medical training.

The nurse handed me the standard paper robe, told me to get undressed, and then left. Maria put all my clothes in a plastic bag; she'd have them ready for me when it would be time to leave the hospital.

Shortly after I'd changed, two young men came in and introduced themselves as my anesthesiologists. It seemed a little odd to me that two guys were needed for the job, but I didn't say anything. They asked if they should get a wheel chair to bring me to the operating room.

I said, "No thanks, I'll walk the last mile."

I looked at Maria and the two gas passers. No one seemed to appreciate my sense of humor this early in the morning, and so Maria and I walked down the hall hand-in-hand. The two anesthesiologists were right behind us. Less than a minute later, we arrived at the OR's big double doors.

I said, "See ya later, babe."

I kissed and hugged my wife and then walked into the operating room, trying hard not to look nervous.

There were about a half dozen people already in the room when I entered. Dr. S was there and greeted me with a big smile. He asked me how I felt. I told him that I felt fine, and that I'd like to go on feeling that way. This time there were chuckles, which made me feel a little better. The surgical robot was a few feet away. It looked like a big metal spider. I hate spiders. Dr. S said they called it "George."

The anesthesiologist twins moved me over to the operating table and told me to lie down. One threw a sheet over me while the other moved some equipment over toward me. Before I knew it, he had a needle in my arm. Dr. S asked if I had any questions. I asked him if "George" had been recently calibrated. He seemed to like that—I think. I don't remember much after that until I woke up.

The Morning After

Let me say right now that post-prostatectomy recovery is, very literally, a pain in the ass. This should come as no big surprise. That digital rectal exam you looked forward to at your annual physical is a big hint why. The prostate is located right next to the rectum, within easy reach of that probing index finger. So when your smiling surgeon removes your prostate, your rectum is going to be somewhat sensitive for a period of time. Fortunately, you'll get medication that can help you to get through this.

The nerve-sparing robotic procedure left me with about a half-dozen small stitched-up openings around a swollen belly from the robotic manipulators that had been dancing around in my innards. One of the pluses to this type of surgery is that you wind up with these little scars that fade with time, instead of one big scar marking the space between your belly button and your pecker.

When I woke up after the surgery, I reached down under the bed covers to check if the nerve-sparing technique had worked. Sure enough, Mr. Johnson could feel my probing fingers just fine! And there was something else—a plastic tube. It was odd to feel a catheter down there, but for the moment, I was relieved that I wasn't going to go through the rest of my life with numb nuts.

Initially, I could neither sit up nor get out of bed without help. But once I was out of bed, I was able, with the assistance of a very patient nurse, to walk around a bit. The nurse walked with me for a while until I regained my footing. Before too long, I was able to walk on my own with some difficulty. I was still very sore and still under the influence of the hospital's industrial-strength medication, but only a few hours after surgery, I was up and walking around.

My point is that, even though your body has been through a traumatic experience, you'll start to recover as soon as you put yourself to the task of getting better.

Pluses and Minuses

After you wake up from surgery, some things will have been lost, and some things will have been gained. You will no longer have a prostate, seminal vesicles, or the sphincter muscle you've come to depend upon for piss control. You will, however, have a brand-spanking new Foley catheter, complete with a urine bag hanging off the side of your bed.

The Foley catheter is a tube that runs from a plastic bag, up to and through the length of your penis and into your bladder. There are various types of catheter systems. The one that I was fitted with was held secure with a small balloon, inflated with water, to hold it securely in place inside my bladder.

The nice thing about a Foley is that you never have to leave your bed to take a leak. The fluid that would normally collect in your bladder automatically drains into your urine bag. The Foley system is neat and clean and allows your body to pass urine so easily that you generally won't even know it's happening.

But there is a not-so-nice side to the Foley. For one thing, it is a foreign object placed inside what is arguably your body's most sensitive area. The catheter tube itself has weight and limited length, and these can act together to tug on you in uncomfortable ways. The catheter tube installed in me extended about three feet out to a two-liter plastic urine bag. I found that I could reduce the tugging while I was sitting or lying in bed by using the weight of my leg to keep the tube from moving around.

Lesson Learned: Imagine you're lying in bed with the urine bag on your right, pull up a short length of the catheter tube and run it under your right thigh. The weight of your leg will likely be enough to keep the tube from pulling while you sit or lie in bed. The catheter tube is not easily collapsed, and it will remain open even with the weight of your leg on it. I found this to be very helpful when trying to get to sleep.

DO NOT ATTEMPT TO PULL OUT THE CATHETER!

Not only would this be insanely painful, it could cause all manner of urological damage.

Remember that there's a little, non-collapsible balloon inside you holding the catheter in place.
Leave it alone. It'll come out soon enough. Trust me.

Word to the Wise: Stay hydrated. Drink a lot of water. Avoid milk and carbonated drinks. Most juices are probably okay, but check with your doctor. Plain water is the preferred beverage for people recuperating from a prostatectomy.

The Foley's Dark Side: Clogs and Blockages

It's amazing how you can come to miss the simple things in life—like taking a leak when you feel the need. It's even more amazing how painful it can be when you can't take a leak when you really, *really* feel the need.

You have no control when fitted with a Foley. The idea is that fluid flows freely from your bladder into the bag, but your Foley can get clogged. How? The most *unlikely* reason is that you've been fitted with a faulty Foley. Foley catheters are simple and reliable devices—it's a tube and a balloon—not much can go wrong there. Despite this, blood clots and little bits of tissue left over from the surgery can get stuck in the catheter opening and prevent the free flow of urine. The result: your bladder gets stretched to capacity when filled with fluid. Thus, the key to happiness when wearing a Foley is being able to tell if there is a problem *before* it becomes a problem.

Your urine bag has lines printed on the side to give you some idea of how much liquid is in it. Typically, the average guy generates about thirty milliliters of urine per hour. Of course, you may make more, or you might make less. The point is, you have a way to tell if you're not passing urine regularly. If it turns out you are falling short in pee-pee production, you may have a clogged Foley and you should take *immediate* action to correct it.

A doctor or nurse can perform a very simple and painless procedure when a Foley blockage occurs. It is called "irrigating the Foley." Although this is a simple procedure, it should only be performed by people who have been trained to do it. Remember, you just got out of surgery, and you are especially vulnerable to infection, so let the people who are experienced in these matters help you. And don't be shy about asking for help!

Irrigating the Foley consists of:

- Detaching the urine bag
- Attaching a large plastic syringe containing a sterile saline solution to where the urine bag was connected
- Injecting the sterile saline solution into the bladder through the Foley catheter

This might sound scary but there's really nothing to it. There is no piercing of the skin. The syringe attaches to the catheter, which is already installed.

Irrigating the Foley is really nothing more than reversing the flow of liquid through the catheter, using sterile saline solution to push the nasty bits blocking the opening back into the bladder. The nurse will then pull some liquid out of the bladder with the syringe. If the blockage was caused by bits of tissue or blood clots, they will likely show up inside the syringe.

This procedure is not painful, but you may feel some strange sensations while it's being done. After the syringe is removed, the urine bag is then reattached and voila! You are now literally good to go! Your Foley may have to be irrigated a few times within the first few days of your recovery. I had to have it done twice after I woke up after the surgery and then twice again after I got home.

Back at home, about a day after the surgery, I began to feel very uncomfortable down below. It was in the middle of the night, and I noticed that the fluid level in my urine bag was low. I tried to bear down gently—but I didn't want to bust anything inside, if you know what I mean. Eventually, the pressure became somewhat painful. Maria called the hospital where I'd had the surgery, some twenty miles away. We were instructed to go to the nearest hospital, less than five miles away, so my wife and I rushed to the emergency room and waited a short agonizing eternity before a nurse came by to irrigate my Foley. The procedure took five minutes, and afterward, I was a new man!

Late the next morning, I noticed that I hadn't filled the urine bag overnight as expected. I wasn't in any pain; I wasn't even uncomfortable. And so we took a nice calm trip back to the hospital. I casually read a magazine in the emergency room while waiting for a nurse. Sure enough, when the irrigation was performed again, more clots and gooey things came streaming out. After that, I didn't require another irrigation.

One of the guys I talked to about his prostatectomy told me that he never had to have his Foley irrigated, but another guy needed irrigation a number of times. He said that his doctor recommended bearing down hard to clear the catheter. I find the idea of bearing down like that right after surgery is just plain scary. You and your doctor should work out a plan to address what to do if and when your catheter clogs. You should ask your doctor about doing the Foley irrigation yourself or have someone else at home do it for you. It's an easy procedure to learn, but because you are actively injecting fluid into your body so soon after surgery, the risk of infection may preclude letting someone without medical training attempt it. Consider how far you are from an emergency room as part of the decision as to whether or not you should perform your own irrigations.

It's important to remember to monitor your urine level throughout the course of the day and especially in the morning when you wake up. If you're not filling your urine bag, don't wait until the last minute to call your doctor. You may need irrigation, or you may have something called a "spastic bladder." Apparently, the bladder itself can prevent urine from flowing into the catheter. I don't understand how this can happen with a tube inserted up there, but there is medication to help prevent it. Here's the bottom line: if you're not filling the bag, call the doctor.

Lesson Learned:

Don't let your bladder fill up while wearing a Foley because it will hurt like hell and make you miserable. Monitor your urine level throughout the day. If you don't seem to be passing enough urine, call your doctor right away.

Silent But (Feels) Deadly

Another source of pain comes from not being able to pass gas. I suffered with this the day after surgery, and it took more than a week before I could fart like a normal person again. Why wasn't I able to pass gas? Probably because of the intestinal swelling in the area where my prostate was removed.

As kids we used to laugh about what could happen to you if you "held it in" for too long. Today, I can tell you what happens—it hurts. And it sucks. But I was warned about this, so I bought a box of anti-gas chewable tablets. When I realized what was going on, I took a couple of these tablets. They worked fast and they worked well. I never thought that I'd miss farting so much! It is, indeed, the little things in life that make it worth living.

The Wonderful Rubber Ring

The prostatectomy also left me with a minor hemorrhoid problem. I don't know why hemorrhoids had to make an appearance at this particular time, perhaps it's just part of my charm. I say "minor," but anyone who has experienced swollen hemorrhoids knows that they feel anything but minor when you have to put up with them.

The usual remedies apply here. In my case, I used medicated wipes to help bring down the swelling, and I sat on a standard inflatable rubber ring, available from almost any drug store. It took about a month for my posterior to regain 'roid composure. My hemorrhoids were more or less a minor inconvenience when compared with the other nasties I had to deal with from the surgery, but they were a literal pain in the ass nonetheless, and I was very happy to have that rubber ring around.

More Fun with Foley: Cleanliness Is Happiness

Guys, we're all aware that Mr. Johnson will grow and shrink throughout the day, depending upon such things as temperature, physical activity, daydreams, or even the people we meet. This doesn't change much when a Foley is installed. The difference is that the Foley catheter doesn't change length—ever. What this means is that your penis is going to slide up and down the catheter tube throughout the course of the day. When it does, the inside of your urethra will deposit a thin trace of mucus on the outside of the catheter tube. This mucus will dry and harden when it's exposed to air. The result: the outside of the catheter is transformed from a nice, smooth, plastic surface to something akin to sandpaper.

The trick is to keep the catheter as clean as possible. I got into the habit of taking a quick shower several times a day just to ensure that my Foley catheter was nice and clean. In addition, an over-the-counter antibacterial ointment can be applied to the catheter near the penis opening to reduce irritation.

Lesson Learned: Discuss in detail with your doctor the best way to handle keeping your catheter clean and the possible use of ointments.

Hangin' with Your Foley

Hospital beds are geared up for any number of contingencies, and they're remarkably adjustable. They go up, they go down, they roll, and they have places on them to hang lots of things, including urine bags. But now you've come home, and you're going to sleep in your own bed. Strangely enough, most home beds aren't built with urine bags in mind. So how and where are you supposed to hang your urine bag while trying to get a good night's sleep? You must be sure to keep the urine bag below your waist at all times, and letting it just lie on the floor while you're in bed is just not a good idea. Suppose it started to leak? What if someone stepped on it? Your Foley hookup is air-tight, or should be—stepping on the urine bag might force used pee inside of thee. Yuk.

My solution was to use a clothes hanger. I slid the hanger between the box spring and the mattress, leaving a corner of the hanger sticking out about an inch. Voila! The hook on my Foley bag now had a place to rest while I slept. I placed the hanger along the length of the bed about midway between where my knees and feet would be when I was lying down (remembering to place the catheter tube underneath my leg so it wouldn't tug on poor Mr. Johnson). The bag was now within easy reach when I got out of bed, and there are no sharp edges on which to accidentally hurt myself or anyone passing by. If you have visitors, you can drape the bedcovers over the bag (just in case you're concerned about such things).

And talking about getting in and out of bed, I generally needed help to do this until about three or four days after the surgery. My gut was swollen and sensitive, and it hurt to try to sit up. I found it to be less painful when getting out of bed by lying on my side and using my legs to rotate my body until they were off the side of the bed. Once my feet were on the floor, I didn't have to bend quite so much to get out of bed. Usually I'd just wimp out and call for help.

Hands-Free Technology

Before there were hands-free cell phones, there was the strap-on urine bag, which is a small plastic bag, maybe half the size of the main bag you woke up with, which straps onto one of your thighs. Sweat pants or other loose-fitting clothing can make it appear as though you're not even wearing a Foley.

Although the strap-on urine bag can be a virtual godsend in terms of mobility, there are a few things to keep in mind when using them.

- Don't cross your legs. You never want the urine bag to be at or above the same level as your bladder. Remember, you've just gotten out of surgery, and you must guard yourself against anything that might lead to infection.

The last thing you need is for stale urine to flow from your Foley bag *back* into your bladder!

- Don't lie on the floor.
- Don't recline in reclining chairs.
- Avoid handstands and cartwheels.
- In short, always keep your Foley bag *below* your waistline.

A Few Foley Tips:

- If you're like me and like to lie on the couch while watching TV, make sure that the Foley bag is strapped below the knee. You can now lie back on the couch with the foot of the "Foley leg" on the floor, ensuring that the bag stays below your waist.

- Let your manhood hang. Position the bag on your leg so that the catheter tube hangs freely from your penis. You don't want the catheter to tug in any direction, as this can cause chafing, which is bound to make you somewhat cranky.

- As mentioned before, cleanliness is happiness. When your leg moves, the catheter moves. You can take steps to reduce how much it moves, but move it will. The cleaner the catheter tube, the happier you will be.

- Finally, check the bag every once in a while. It's surprising how fast that small bag can fill up. Again, you want to minimize the possibility of old urine backing up into the bladder.

Walking with Foley

Walking, as it turns out, is a very important component of recovery. As soon as you have your newfound freedom, thanks to the strap-on urine bag, you should make a point of walking around a lot. Discuss a daily walking regiment with your doctor and stick to it. Walking is one of those wonderful things that doesn't cost anything to do, yet it can work wonders for your recovery.

But be warned, walking around with a Foley can be ... interesting. Before going for a walk, make sure your catheter tube is clean (Mr. Johnson hates the sandpaper slide) and ensure that it's adjusted for minimum motion.

I like to walk, and after an extended session, my urine would run a little pink and I'd get some blood seeping outside the catheter tube. When this happened, I would take a shower to clean up, paying special attention to cleaning the catheter tube. I'd then take it easy the rest of the day and be a little less aggressive in my walk the following day.

Walking after surgery is important, but you don't want to get so aggressive that you injure yourself. This is yet another topic you should discuss with your doctor.

Switching Urine Bags: Simple, But Not To Be Taken Lightly

When it comes time to switch from your large, overnight bag to the smaller travel size, or vice versa, it is very important that you take special care not to compromise the overall sterility of your catheter system. Remember, you are especially sensitive to infection after surgery. When changing from one bag to another, take the time to do it right. Here are the general steps I used:

1. Clean the tube connector of the bag that you want to attach with a fresh alcohol wipe and place it to one side, taking care that the connector does not touch any surrounding items. After cleaning the connector, wrap it inside the wrapper that the alcohol wipe came out of. After all, the inside of the wrapper has got to be as germ-free as the wipe itself.

2. Disconnect the catheter connection to the urine bag you are currently using. You probably want to

be standing over the toilet when you do this, as you never know when you're about to let loose with a few drips or more.

3. Clean the connector of the tube leading into your bladder with a fresh alcohol wipe, then connect the new urine bag's connector to your catheter, and once again you're good to go!

Before you leave the hospital after surgery, be sure to go through this little procedure with your doctor or nurse, and make sure that you completely understand every step of this simple procedure so that you can perform it easily by yourself.

Parting Is Such Sweet Sorrow

The big day finally arrived: my Foley was going to be removed! The novelty of wearing a Foley faded for me after the first few hours of having to deal with it. After that, I couldn't wait to be rid of the damned thing.

Prior to removing the Foley, the good doctor injected some sterile saline solution into my bladder, then gave me a urine bottle to hold in front of me so his hands were free to do what he had to do. Removal of the catheter was no big deal. I stood in front of the doctor as he deflated the little balloon that kept the catheter in place.

Then he said, "On the count of three. One, two ..." He gave a quick tug, and it slid right out. "Three."

I felt no pain, but I did briefly feel some unusual pressure. It didn't tickle, it didn't hurt—it was just strange. Immediately after the tube was removed, I was urinating. There was a mild burning sensation as urine flowed freely, but that passed quickly. The doc asked me to try to stop the flow. I was able to bear down and stop it, and then he told me to let it all out.

The trick I now had to learn was to regain my control over urinating. This is not nearly as easy as it sounds. When guys grow up, we unconsciously learn to use the sphincter muscle in the prostate to control urine flow. Those muscles were removed with the prostate. Fortunately, there is another muscle near the base of the urinary bladder that we can learn to use to control urine flow. Learning this takes time. Ask any two-year-old girl.

Permission to Wet Your Pants: Granted

Until we master our new golden-flow control, we get to wear disposable underwear, diapers, and pads. In short, we're going to wind up wetting our pants for a while and will have to live for a time with a continually wet crotch. This isn't as much fun as it sounds. The situation may be a bit more bearable for guys who have retained their foreskin. But us circumcised guys will have the most sensitive parts of our manhood continually in contact with the cold, damp fabric of our absorbent undergarment. I found the chafing uncomfortable and distracting. You might consider covering Mr. Johnson's bald head with an ample amount of Vaseline® to protect it from the damp surface of your undergarment of choice.

I found adult diapers very uncomfortable, but absorbent underwear and pads were definitely preferable. None of these absorbent undergarments are as comfortable as regular underwear. When it comes to my crotch, I'm all about comfort, so I had a real incentive to regain control of my urinary functions. I started working at it the day the catheter was removed. What the heck, I needed a hobby anyway.

At the time I'm writing this part of this book, about four months after my surgery, I've gone from using four or five absorbent underpants per day to a single absorbent pad per day, and the pad is almost completely dry by the time I remove it at day's end.

Below is a summary of the absorbent undergarments I've tried. It's probably due to my Scottish heritage that I have a problem using my hard-earned money to pay for something, piss in it for a while, and then throw it away. I don't like pissing my money away. You might do a little research at local pharmacies and retail stores to find the best prices for absorbent undergarments. I checked out purchasing this stuff online, but I found that the online prices, even when shipping was "free," were more expensive than what I could find locally. It seems that one pays for the convenience of home delivery.

Disposable Underwear:

- Comfortable and quiet
- Two or more per day initially
- The most expensive of the three types of garments I've tried; purchased in a package of sixteen or eighteen

Diapers:

- Less expensive than disposable underwear
- Not nearly as comfortable as disposable underwear or pads
- Makes an annoying and potentially embarrassing *swishing* sound when you move
- Purchase in a package of sixteen or eighteen

Pads

- Small, comfortable, and silent
- Used with most snug underwear, tighty whities preferred
- Lacks the capacity of disposable underwear or diapers
- Cheapest of the three, but may need several (three to six) when first used
- Purchase in packages of fifty

For the first month, I used the disposable underwear. When I got down to using only one a day, I switched to using pads. The number of pads you use in a day reflects the extent of your control. I was very encouraged the day I realized that I had used only two pads. Little things can mean a lot.

Personal note: The first time I purchased adult diapers, I felt a little self-conscious. The cashier and the folks behind me could all see what I was buying. The cashier didn't say anything, but the smirk on his face pretty much gave away what he was thinking. I shrugged and told him I was stocking up for the Super Bowl: "We don't want to miss a thing!"

Now, as lame as this sounds, it got a chuckle out of the cashier. But we all laughed when the guy wearing a Teamster's cap in back of me exclaimed, "Hey, that's a good idea!"

A Certain Air about You?

Here's a fact a life: if you consistently piss in the same place, that place will eventually smell like piss. Henceforth, we shall refer to this axiom as Johnson's Rule.

Absorbent undergarments are bound to acquire the scent of their contents in accordance with Johnson's Rule. But don't worry; there are a few simple things you can do to keep from smelling like a gas station urinal.

- *Always* make the effort of using the toilet instead of relying on your underwear. The absorbency of your underwear is to save you from accidents. It is *not* a replacement for the commode!
- Change your undergarment when you get a whiff of that unmistakable scent. The use of pads makes this easy.
- Apply a light sprinkle of talcum powder. Talcum also has the benefit of reducing chafing.
- Avoid eating asparagus or any other food that provides an embellishment to your natural territorial-marking fragrance.
- If you *want* to be left alone, you don't have anything to worry about. Just ignore the previous four bullet points.

I was dismayed early on in my use of absorbent undergarments when I could detect the scent of urine following me around wherever I went, but I discovered two things: first, people had to get very close to me to smell what I could smell. Whenever I could smell it and whenever possible, I took a quick, hot rinse in the shower before changing undergarments. The second thing was that the prospect of stinking like piss provided me with even more incentive to regain control over my bladder, and it turns out that Kegel exercises are the key to that control.

Kegel Exercises

Kegel exercises are all important in helping you strengthen and control the group of muscles (sometimes referred to as the PC muscles) in your pelvic floor. The urethra passes through the pelvic floor, so it makes sense that the more control you're able to exert over these muscles, the better you'll be able to control urine flow.

Exercising pelvic floor muscles is pretty simple:

1. Squeeze the pelvic floor for ten seconds
2. Relax the pelvic floor muscles for ten seconds
3. Repeat steps 1 and 2 ten times

And that's all there is to it. Do this three times a day, morning, noon, and night. It takes a little over three minutes to do this simple workout, and because these muscles are *inside* your body, you can do them anywhere you want without attracting attention.

When you first start doing Kegel exercises, you may have a problem isolating the proper muscles down there. Do not clench your thigh muscles or your buttocks. It's a good idea to try to keep these muscles relaxed when doing Kegel exercises. One way to isolate the pelvic floor muscles is while standing and trying to flex these muscles, you should see your penis move slightly. This is an indication that you've got the right group of muscles isolated for Kegel work. These are the same muscles you would use to maintain an erection.

Another way to isolate this muscle group is to sit on the toilet and start urinating. Then try stopping the flow. I suggest sitting on the toilet because you're not going to have the control you used to have. By sitting on the toilet you're less likely to decorate the surrounding area with processed beverages.

Initially when you start Kegel exercises, you may find it difficult to squeeze for a full ten seconds. Don't sweat it. Squeeze and relax for one or two seconds to start. Improvement comes quickly. Before you know it, squeezing and holding for ten seconds will become easy.

I've read that "flexing" pelvic floor muscles fast and hard doesn't really help control urine flow because the muscles become fatigued. The result is that leakage can occur more easily. Slow and steady wins the race. My surgeon recommended the ten-second method and it's worked very well for me.

How long will it be before you're back to normal? About five weeks into my recovery, I was just getting around to trying pads, a significant improvement over needing the higher-capacity absorbent underwear. It took a little over a month for me to go from being completely "diaper dependent" to requiring a urine pad in the event of an accident. I understand that some patients are told to start doing kegel exercises a few weeks prior to surgery. Apparently the idea is to develop the PC muscles and shorten the period of incontinence after the Foley catheter is removed.

The day that my Foley came out, I was completely incontinent and I discovered the hard way that the pad wasn't enough to handle my needs at the time.

Out On My Own Again

It was November 13, 2009, at 9:00 AM. My appointment to get de-Foleyed. When the catheter was finally removed, I felt as though I was set free from a leash! The catheter was gone, and Mr. Johnson was swingin' on his own again!

The doc seemed surprised that I had only brought a pad with me instead of a diaper or absorbent underwear, but he patiently showed me how to set up the pad in my tighty whities. By the time I arrived back home, I had to get to the bathroom right away. When I got out of the car, I felt a squirt come out, but I was able to stop it with some effort. Despite my unexpected leakage, I was relieved that my pants and underwear were still dry, thanks to the pad.

With my wife at work, I was home alone and feeling good. No more Foley! I was getting antsy hanging around the house, but it was too cold outside to go for a walk. There were a lot of chores I might have done, but I was forbidden from lifting anything. Then a commercial for the movie *2012* appeared on TV. It was opening today, at a theater near me! Now, I'm a big science fiction fan. It had been a couple of hours since the doc removed the Foley, and I had to hit the head only once in all that time. After thinking about how absorbent the pads seemed to be, I decided *What the hell, let's go to the movies!*

I changed the pad, not because it was full but because I wanted to leave the house with a fresh, empty one. I grabbed my trusty, inflatable, red-rubber ring and drove out to the theater.

Driving while sitting on the rubber ring was not a big problem after I adjusted the car seat. At the movie-theater parking lot, the cold triggered another squirt when I got out of the car, but there wasn't much to it and the pad I was wearing did its job with ease. Once in the theater, I had a little bit of difficulty standing on line for a while. It had only been eight days since the prostatectomy. I was still stiff and a bit sore from the surgery but it wasn't bad enough to make me turn around and go home. I bought the ticket, passed right by the concession stand, and headed straight for the men's room. I wanted to start the show with an empty bladder just to be on the safe side.

I found an aisle seat just before the show started. Again, I wanted to be on the safe side. I didn't want to have to pass in front of a lot of people in case of an emergency bathroom break. Sitting on the rubber ring and reclining in the theater chair actually felt kind of cozy. I hadn't been this comfortable in a long time (actually, it was only a little more than a week, but it felt like forever). The lights went down, and the show started. I enjoyed the movie thoroughly—the ending seemed a little bit hokey, but never mind! I sat through almost two hours of a sci-fi action flick without the need to pee! Fantastic! If this kept up I'd be back to work in a week!

The lights came up, and I stood up. That's when I suddenly realized that my wonderful inflatable rubber ring, the pliant device that made sitting possible by contouring its shape to match my bottom so precisely, had actually applied enough pressure to my pelvic floor to prevent fluid from passing through my urethra. In short, my bladder had been filling up all during the two-hour movie. When I stood up, it was like opening the floodgates. It was as if someone had poured a warm bucket of water down the front of my pants—*right there in the movie theater.* The pad I was wearing was no match for the pent-up pee-pee pressure.

I cannot adequately express the profound sense of surprise, embarrassment, and frustration I felt at that moment. It was the first time in more than half a century that I had publicly pissed my pants.

Even more surprising was the fact that no one seemed to notice!

When the lights came up, the crowd in the theater began pushing to leave. I was wearing black sweat pants and a long winter coat. If anyone looked at me at all, it was because I was carrying a red rubber ring. As I rushed out of the theater, the warm urine covering my legs suddenly turned icy cold. When I got to my car, I threw an old tarp from the trunk over the driver's seat, put the rubber ring on top of that, carefully positioned myself on top of the ring, and drove home. After a shower and a change of clothes—including a fresh pair of absorbent underwear, not a pad—I was okay.

In hindsight, I can't believe that I was actually dumb enough to go to the movies just hours after my catheter had been removed. But then, I felt so good to finally be free from my friend Foley that I thought I could do almost anything. I was wrong.

I purchased more disposable absorbent underwear that day and went through three or four of them before bedtime. I also wore them to bed. I have to admit, I am impressed by the amount of fluid those diapers can absorb.

Lesson Learned: In the words of Dirty Harry, "A man's got to know his limitations." Don't overestimate your abilities after surgery. At the very least, you might embarrass yourself. At worst, you might seriously injure yourself.

A Man of Many Colors

Before the prostatectomy, my urine was clear or slightly yellow. After surgery, as one might expect, plenty of red and pink made appearances at tinkle time.

I was prescribed a drug to help prevent urinary infections after the Foley was removed. While on this prescription, my urine turned green and blue! It turns out this is normal. There was no pain associated with the color change, but be aware that this pretty color will stain any fabric it comes into contact with (as evidenced by my formally white tighty whities).

A few days after the prescription was completed, I resumed my normal golden flow. My undies, however, still bear a slight bluish tinge after months of washings.

I'm a Big Boy Now!

About four weeks after the Foley was removed, I noticed when I got out of bed that my absorbent underwear wasn't filling up very much, but when I stood, it was another matter. I'd struggle for control as I rushed for the toilet. After some effort over the next few days I found that it became easier to hold my water until I got to the bathroom and piss in the way I remembered an early morning piss used to be.

It was a supremely satisfying experience.

I became confident enough to try wearing tighty whities and a pad to bed. The next morning, the pad had done its work, but it was nowhere near filled to capacity. It was as if I'd had one or two minor leaks, and that was it. A week later, I had grown confident enough to try not wearing any sort of absorbent underwear to bed. I still had to get up in the middle of the night, maybe two to three hours after going to bed, to take a leak. For a couple of weeks more, I had to get up more than once during the night, but the upside was that I didn't have to wear special underwear to keep my bed dry.

About nine weeks after the surgery, I started to sleep straight through the night. However, when I got out of bed in the morning, the main priority was getting to the toilet.

Wrest Easy

It was the second or third night of not using absorbent underwear to bed that I, after more than fifty years, actually wet the bed. I remember dreaming that I was standing in front of a urinal when I suddenly woke up and realized that I wasn't even close to a urinal. Fortunately, Maria had anticipated this possibility and had padded my side of the bed.

I was mortified, and I felt a little ashamed. But really, all it took to set things right was a change of sheets and a late-night shower. After an impromptu wash day for the soiled sheets, there was no evidence that I had relived a moment from my childhood.

Despite this embarrassing enuretic episode, I felt that I had to draw a line in the sand. I realized that if I wanted to sleep through the night, I'd have to work at it. I had to be willing to have accidents in order to succeed. So I decided *not* to wear absorbent underwear the very next night. The bed's been dry ever since.

I'm telling you this so that you know there can be surprises, and that when there are surprises, it's best to just take them in stride and keep your focus on the goal. In my humble opinion, you have to focus on your successes more than your failures during recovery.

To Push or Not to Push

When I woke up after prostate surgery, I was completely incontinent. Four months later, I find myself sometimes having to *bear down* to get a flow going. It's easy to get into the habit of pushing to piss. However, very often, all I have to do to get the golden flow streaming is relax. The Kegel exercises have given me control over those PC muscles. If you find yourself unable to perform at the urinal, don't panic. Just relax and wait and let Mother Nature and gravity take control.

Challenging Times: The Sneak Leak

As I write this, it's been almost sixteen weeks since my surgery, and although I have improved considerably, I still don't have complete flow control all day long. On occasion, a small, unexpected squirt gets by the gate. The pad I wear makes this a non-issue. When it happens, the only one who knows that I took a sneak leak is me.

A sneak leak can happen:

- Standing up after sitting
- While walking
- After any sudden movement
- Coughing, sneezing, or laughing
- Lifting something
- Bending
- Because of an impending bowel movement
- Farting
- Sudden temperature changes (going outside when it's cold)

You may experience a squirt once or twice while you're just standing around doing nothing. I've found that this generally means it was time to empty the bladder. It seems to me that the prostate probably provides a signal to the brain, letting it know there's pressure building in the bladder and we unconsciously interpret this as a need to seek out a nearby urinal or tree. Without a prostate to provide this subtle signal, our body has to learn to deal with its new set of plumbing arrangements. It takes time to learn new habits.

It's Clench Time!

Having experienced more sneak leaks than I'd like to admit since the surgery, I've taken to "clenching down" just before I attempt to lift something, or just before standing after sitting . I'm attempting to learn and internalize a new behavior at the ripe old age of fifty-five. My hope is that, if I do this every time I even suspect a sneak leak might occur and if I do it long enough, it will become an unconscious habit. I'll clench down automatically without thinking about it, and I'll eventually put a stop to the sneak leak.

Going Commando

About three months after the surgery, I started to go without a pad at home. I still wore normal underwear, but around the house, I tried to work without a net. It seemed to me that as long as I knew the pad was there, I knew it would be okay to let a squirt get by the gate. I wanted to get back to the point to where I didn't need a pad at all. So far, I've been fairly successful. There have been minor slipups from time to time, and I know it's going to take a while, but that's okay. I'll take the time I need in order to get what I want.

Prior to the surgery, I would typically hit the head maybe two or three times during the course of the day. These days, I make that trip almost twice as much. I've become an opportunistic pisser, visiting the urinal not necessarily because I have to go but because I have an opportunity to empty the bladder. To be sure, I can hold my water as well as the next guy thanks to those Kegel exercises. But there are those times, such as after sitting for a while or doing something suddenly strenuous, that a sneak leak might occur. The less urine I carry around with me, the lower the likelihood that I'll have a sneak leak when I let my guard down.

Number Two on my List of Concerns: Low Resi-Doodoo

Before I could be released from the hospital, I was required to have a bowel movement. I was able to squeeze one out (a little one; it barely qualified), and it was tough, and I then had to deal with constipation issues for the next five or six weeks. The pain from delayed dumping was minimal compared with not being able to piss or fart, but it was still very uncomfortable.

Immediately after surgery, I was placed on what is referred to as a "low-residue" diet. The surgeon, in removing my prostate, worked very close to the rectum, so it seemed prudent to avoid performing any "heavy-doody" off-loading for a while. As it happened, even the results of the low-residue diet gave me some trouble when assuming *The Thinker* position on the porcelain throne.

I've provided an example of a low-residue diet in an appendix of this book for reference. Be sure to discuss your post-surgery dietary requirements with your doctor.

Medication—a Mixed Blessing

After surgery, I was initially prescribed a fairly powerful pain killer. A few weeks later, my pain medication was changed, but it was just as potent. Though both of these miracles of modern medicine made my post-surgical pain bearable, using them came with a price. Both medications have a potential side effect: they can cause constipation in some patients and lucky me, I was one of them. So, on the one hand, I was relieved from the pain of surgery, but on the other hand, I was hampered by the discomfort of not being able to take a decent dump. Walking helped the situation somewhat, and I took a stool softener on a daily basis. From time to time, I had to take a laxative to keep things moving along.

As the intensity of the post-surgery pain began to decline, I started taking my pain medication on an as-needed basis only, being careful never to exceed the recommended dosage. I wanted to get away from taking the pills altogether so that I could get back on a regular schedule. Three weeks after surgery, the discomfort had decreased to the point that taking Ibuprofen was just as effective at relieving my pain as the prescribed drugs, and my "bottom line" activity was slowly returning to normal.

I was advised by my doctor to take laxatives two or three times over the month and a half after my surgery. Most laxatives, in my opinion, taste a great deal like the stuff they're supposed to move, so after more than a month of on-again-off-again constipation, I decided on my own to try something my grandmother told us kids about when I was little.

"Drink your prune juice," she would say, and so I did. And for me, the prune juice worked better than the laxatives. And it tasted a whole lot better too! The morning BM from drinking a tall glass of prune juice the night before produced a monster compared with the results from using laxatives, and it was relatively easy to pass. Again, I felt I had passed a major milestone … in more ways than one.

Note: I decided to try the prune juice approach more than a month after my surgery, and *after* my doctor advised me that it was all right to go off the low-residue diet.

Lesson Learned: Sometimes the good old-fashioned ways work the best. For me, a brisk walk, prune juice, and fruit worked wonders, but remember to discuss any dietary or medicinal changes you are considering with your doctor *before* you make them.

The BIG Question

It's the question all guys will all ask: will it ever get hard again? From what I understand, if you were having problems getting it up prior to surgery, a prostatectomy isn't going to restore your ability.

Ten months after the surgery, I hadn't realized the final answer to this question. Only about 20 percent of prostatectomy patients do not have erection problems after radical prostatectomy. I'm not one of those 20 percent. I'm one of the 80 percent who have to wait and see if there's wood in their future. In fact, the first few weeks after surgery, it seemed that Mr. Johnson was attempting to withdraw *inside* my body. The poor guy—he was in shock.

From what I've read, there is a chance that my love lance will stand straight and tall once again. Some 75 percent of guys younger than sixty (that would be me) eventually regain rigidity to some extent. A full recovery can take months, a year, or more in many cases.

During the first few months of my recovery, while performing Kegel exercises, I could sometimes feel the familiar sensations that used to accompany an erection, and sure enough, there were indications that the flesh was willing. Two months after surgery, I had yet to attain anything resembling my former glory. Four months after surgery, there was noticeable improvement, but there was quite a way to go before I would have my towel hanger back. Some doctors encourage patients to continually try to obtain an erection. Apparently, just trying can aid in recovery. Well, okay. If I *have* to.

Medication typically used to treat erectile dysfunction was prescribed for me as soon as I left the hospital. Apparently, an increased blood flow in the affected region can speed repair down there, and that's bound to entice Mr. Johnson to stand up and take notice.

However, the reality is that even by diligently taking your medication there still remains the possibility that you may need a pill, injection, urethral suppository or some other means to obtain and maintain an erection. It seems that losing the capability to obtain an erection on your own is the risk you take when dealing with prostate cancer, regardless of how you choose to do it.

And as if that weren't enough, there is an ongoing controversy about whether or not prostate surgery and other therapies can permanently affect the length and size of your love muscle. Part of the problem in clarifying this issue stems from the lack of clinical data. No doctor I've ever visited has asked me how tall Mr. Johnson stood. Measuring the size of an erect penis is not typically a part of a routine physical. And really, unless they're hung like a Clydesdale, what are the chances that guys are going to be completely honest when asked the question?

In point of fact, almost a year after undergoing prostatectomy surgery, my Willie has the will, but not the stature he used to have. What I had become accustomed to thinking of as a handful is not as much as it used to be.

In my humble opinion, when it comes down to choosing between risking a slow, agonizing death from prostate cancer, or living with a stunted or slouching penis, Mr. Johnson takes second place. In the meantime, ED medication does help my old fella rise to the occasion when called upon.

And, while we're on the subject, yes, you can still experience orgasm. It's just a lot drier than it used to be. If the cost of never having to live with prostate cancer is shooting blanks, I'm happy to pay it.

Take Your Medicine—If You Can

At the first follow-up visit after surgery, Dr. S provided me with a prescription for a popular blue pill that became very well known for helping men with erectile dysfunction or ED. The prescription was actually for one-fourth of the pill to be taken daily. The purpose of this prescription was to help speed recovery from surgery by enhancing blood flow to the affected areas. Dr. S provided me with eight pills when I left the hospital, enough samples to cover me for a little more than a month.

Later, he switched me to another popular pill. This time, he provided enough samples for a couple of weeks, the strategy was to use my prescription insurance plan to obtain more of the prescription as needed. The problem was that my prescription plan would not provide the quantity of pills prescribed by the surgeon. There was a monthly limit to the amount of ED medication that clients can get through the plan I was paying into. I wound up missing my daily dosage for a time and then ultimately had to pay out of pocket for the balance of the prescription not covered by my prescription plan.

Eventually, with the help of my urologist, an appeal was submitted to my insurance company. The appeal was approved, which covered the cost, minus the co-pay of course, of my prescription. The appeal indicated that the prescription was to help me recover from surgery.

Lesson Learned: If you have insurance that covers the cost of prescription medicines, contact your insurance company to review their policy with respect to ED medications *before* you begin treatment or undergo surgery. If your policy does not provide the quantities of medication that your surgeon will prescribe, the surgeon may be able to submit an appeal. The last thing you need during your recovery is a last-minute misunderstanding with your insurance company that might interrupt your medication schedule and ultimately affect your recovery.

The New Quarterly Review

Every three months after surgery, guys who have undergone a radical prostatectomy subject themselves to a periodic blood test. The test looks for traces of PSA. There is always the chance, no matter how small, that the well-meaning surgeon may have missed a cell or two from the prostate while remodeling your innards. All the people I've spoken to, with one exception, who had a prostatectomy have had their PSA tests come back "undetectable" (they don't like to say zero. If there's PSA in the blood, the test can't find it). Undetectable levels of PSA are a good indication that the surgeon got everything.

But what if the test comes back indicating a tiny level of PSA is still present? That would suggest that there were still at least a few prostate cells still lingering around down there. Or, cells being the tiny things that they are, may have drifted somewhere else in the body.

I'm certainly no medical expert, but I'd imagine that if my PSA test results came back with a number attached, I'd be more surprised than shocked. If this happened, I suspect that my urologist would want to embark on some level of watchful waiting; perhaps increase the frequency of PSA tests to see if there's any substantial change over a short period of time. Remember, not all the cells in your prostate were cancerous. Whatever was left over from the surgery might just be hangin' loose and basking in solitude. The one guy I spoke to that had detectable PSA in his blood after his prostate was removed was something of a special case. For starters, his prostate was abnormally small. He also underwent a number of prostate biopsies before the decision was made to remove it. This one guy wound up getting chemo for a short while as well because his PSA number was still climbing after his prostate was removed. Despite the complication in his special case, the last I'd heard he was doing just fine.

If my PSA level climbed rapidly after surgery, I would certainly consider making use of those therapies that I previously rejected, not because I might have made a mistake with selecting prostatectomy, but because I would *still have the option* to use those other therapies.

As I write this, I've just completed my third PSA "follow-up" test and my PSA level remains undetectable. If all goes well and my next PSA falls in line with the preceding three, I'll only need a PSA test every six months, twice a year for five years. After that it becomes an annual test, just like in the good old days before the surgery.

In Closing

I've attempted to provide a description, in a somewhat light-hearted fashion, of my experiences with radical prostatectomy surgery. I've explained my understanding of the available therapies which led me to choose surgery, as well as my experiences during my recovery. I can assure you that this light-heartedness stems from hindsight. I got through it all okay and I'm feeling fine.

I'd be lying if I didn't tell you that there were a few times during my recovery that were very difficult to get through. All I can suggest to the guys recovering from surgery is to hunker down and tough it out. Try to sleep through it, get involved in a conversation, read a book, watch TV, anything to divert your attention. During those tough times, I'd remember the guys I had talked to who had already been through it all. Just knowing that they had experienced everything I was going through, and that they had come away from it smiling, helped me to get through it, too.

No one dealing with cancer does so lightly. You are literally faced with a life or death decision and you understand that any decision you make comes with life-long consequences. Fortunately, we live in a time where the chances for recovery from prostate cancer are for most guys excellent.

Having been there and done that, six to eight weeks of recovery time to get back on my feet seems a small price to pay for not having to live with the prostate cancer for the rest of my life. Kegel exercises are part of my daily routine from now on. I actually do them in the car on my way to and from work.

It is my sincere hope that if you have been diagnosed with prostate cancer, you will take the time to consider all of your options carefully and grill your doctor and others who have dealt with this issue. You will probably find that prostate cancer patients are willing to talk about their experiences. And don't be afraid to ask the potentially embarrassing questions. After all, what's a little embarrassment in the face of something as insidious as cancer?

Also remember that medical technology advances quickly these days. Many of the concerns I had about the various therapies in 2009 may no longer be relevant. I encourage you to investigate and discuss all the things I've talked about in this book with your doctor and the others that you care to share your concerns with. It's *YOUR* body and *YOUR* life. No questions are off-limits. Never let anyone convince you otherwise.

I started writing this book about five weeks after undergoing radical prostatectomy surgery. Twelve months later, I can report that I feel great and have pretty much adapted to the changes I've had to make in my life. Incontinence is not problem for me, although I admit that a minor squirt does get past the gate once in a great while but the flow is tiny and not usually noticeable by anyone but me. In fact, it *feels* worse than it is. One advantage, if you can call it an advantage, to not having a prostate is that the actual time needed to take a leak has been noticeably reduced. The prostate safety valve is no longer there to slow the flow.

One last piece of personal information that I'm happy to report: Almost a year to the day after prostatectomy surgery, and without taking ED medication for several days, I woke up with a boner.

In hindsight, my recovery wasn't really all that bad after all. My life has changed in some ways, but I've been able to adapt and today I'm able to joke about it. Here's hoping that your recovery will go better than mine.

Best of Luck,

Craig Johnson

Appendix A: Low-Residue Diet

Beverages

Teas, coffee, carbonated beverages

Avoid milk if not otherwise well tolerated.

Cereals

Farina, grits, cream of wheat, cream of rice, cornmeal, Rice Krispies, corn flakes, Special K, and puffed rice

Avoid oatmeal, Wheatena, whole grain and bran cereals, Cheerios, granola, and all cereals containing coconut, dried fruit or nuts.

Potato and Substitutes

White rice, pasta, white potato and sweet potato without the skin

Avoid potato skins, legumes, brown or wild rice, and whole-grain pasta products.

Meat and Dairy

Tender beef, chicken, fish, lamb, liver, pork, turkey, veal, eggs, cottage cheese, and other mild cheeses

Avoid meat and shellfish with tough connective tissue or gristle. Do not eat luncheon meats or sausage with peppercorns, seeds or casings. Steer clear of dried beans or peas. Avoid cheese if not well tolerated.

Vegetables

Limit to a half-cup per day. Eat well-cooked vegetables without seeds and drink vegetable juices without pulp.

Avoid all raw vegetables, artichokes, beans, corn, pumpkin, and split peas.

Fruits

Fruit juices without pulp as desired, *except* prune juice

Fats

Butter, mild gravy, vegetable oil, cream or half and half, and salad dressing without seeds.

Soups

Creamed soups, broth from bouillon made from allowed ingredients

Avoid all soups with legumes and vegetables.

Desserts

Cakes, candies, cookies and pies made from allowed ingredients. Fruit ices, gelatin, Popsicles and sherbet. Ice cream, pudding, and custard (if tolerated) from allowed ingredients.

Others

Catsup, smooth peanut butter, salt, finely ground spices and herbs, vinegar, mustard, jelly, sugar, and syrup

Avoid whole spices in seed form, such as celery seed, caraway seed, fennel, peppercorn, poppy seed and sesame seed. Do not eat chili sauce, popcorn, fruit jams, and preserves containing seeds.

Appendix B: Craig Johnson's Recovery Time Line

This book started out as a collection of notes which I intended to share with guys I met who were considering prostatectomy surgery. One thing lead to another and I wound up writing this book to share my experiences with all men faced with prostate cancer. I put my notes together based mostly on *what* I had experienced rather than *when* I experienced them. In this Appendix I've provided an approximate chronological listing of the events of my recovery; some dates are embedded in my memory. Most of the dates are approximate. It didn't occur to me until after I started editing the book that I should have marked events on a calendar.

November 2, 2009	Started on a daily antibiotic three days prior to surgery.
November 5, 2009	It's prostatectomy time!
November 6, 2009	Home by late afternoon. Figured out how to deal with the urine bag by the bed issue, then went to bed.
	Started low-residue diet (not that I was all that hungry anyway).
	Started ED medication.
November 7, 2009	Urine bag not filling. Bloated bladder. Rush to emergency room for a Foley irrigation.
November 8, 2009	Notice urine bag not filling again. This time a casual trip to the hospital. It's the last time an irrigation is needed.
November 13, 2009	Foley gets removed! Begin Kegel exercises. Later that same day I piss myself at the movies and come to the conclusion that adult diapers are not an option.
November 14, 2009	Blue piss. I'm a one-man rainbow. Thought about making notes into a book.
	Started making notes about recovery in the event family, friends or acquaintances have to go through the same ordeal.
November 30, 2009	Off low-residue diet, also switching to over the counter pain medication.
December (first week), 2009	Say Hallelujah for prune juice!

December, (second week) 2009	Tried wearing urine pads to bed instead of absorbent underwear. Have to get up once or twice during the night to take leak.
December (third week), 2009	Tried not wearing any protection at all in bed. A couple of nights later... oops.
Early January, 2010	Slept straight through the night. Rush to the toilet in the morning. Notes are turning into a book effort.
Late January/Early February, 2010	Still wearing pads to work, but I take them off at home. Need to wean myself off of having them around.
Mid February, 2010	Mr Johnson shows signs of awakening, but still too weak to stand on his own.
First half of April, 2010	Kegel helps me to keep control fairly well, but the occasional squirt gets past the gate.
Early in May, 2010	Goin' for it. Went to work without urine pads. Mission successful. Opportunistic pissing becomes part of the normal workday.
May - October, 2010	ED medication allows Mr. Johnson to stand up and be noticed.
September - October, 2010	Mr. Johnson stands briefly on his own (and with some effort) without the help of ED medication.
November 6, 2010	Morning Wood!